Chronicling Childhood Cancer:

A Collection of Personal Stories by Children and Teens with Cancer

TRISHA PAUL

Published by MPublishing, an imprint of Michigan Publishing
University of Michigan Library

Cover Design by Rohan Paul

ISBN 978-1-60785-437-1

DEDICATION

For children and teens with cancer

CONTENTS

Foreword vii

Preface ix

1. Lexie 1

2. Mary.. 13

3. William 23

4. Shannon 29

5. Celeste 39

6. Jacob.. 49

7. Tamia.. 53

8. Zoey... 61

9. Christina.. 71

10. Ruben... 75

Writing Activity 79

Tell Your Story..................................... 81

About the Editor................................... 83

FOREWORD

I have had the honor of treating children and young adults with cancer of all ages and backgrounds over the last two decades. During this time, I have been a witness to the well-documented medical advances in childhood cancer therapy. However, the personal journeys behind these successes and failures have largely gone unrecognized.

Narratives in this book chronicle these missing stories. Some of the children featured here are my patients. I thought I knew them well through interactions with them and with their parents in the clinic. After reading their stories, I feel like I am being reintroduced to them. Their accounts have honesty, openness and most importantly, an indomitable spirit from which no one can escape untouched. Each child recounts their story in a unique way. Some children had a lot to say, while others took the quieter approach and let their drawings tell their story. But the results were powerful either way!

Healthcare delivery is greatly becoming technology driven and impersonal. Narratives like these play an important role in reminding healthcare providers, relatives and friends of these children, to respect their individuality and personal wishes while they are fighting a very brave fight against cancer. While we are unlikely to win every fight against cancer, this book reminds us that we are first treating a child, a person, and second, treating a cancer patient. Recognizing individuality and personalizing cancer care should be a goal all healthcare providers strive to achieve.

Besides the courageous young patients whose stories have been chronicled here, one of the most heartening aspects for me personally has been this book's young editor. Over the last five years, she has acquired remarkable wisdom and a listening ability while working with these children. She is an aspiring future pediatric oncologist, which gives me tremendous hope in the ability of future generations of pediatric oncologists. She, along with her colleagues, is entrusted with the task of making sure the voices and stories of these brave children will be heard loud and clear for generations to come.

Rajen Mody, M.D., M.S.
Clinical Director, Pediatric Hematology/Oncology
Associate Professor, Department of Pediatrics
University of Michigan Medical School

PREFACE

For five years, I have spent my Friday evenings in a playroom full of toys and games. As a volunteer at C.S. Mott Children's Hospital, I observed cancer's disruptive nature: the imprisonment of IV poles, the pain of pokes, the side effects of chemotherapy. My interactions with the incredible children and families I met over the years made me increasingly curious about how cancer affects a child. I came to wonder how children understand and cope with this mysterious, complex illness.

In studying literature at the University of Michigan, I realized that medicine is all about people and their personal stories. Narratives of illness—told by patients, families, and health providers—can provide greater insight into experiences of living with diseases like cancer.

We hear stories about children with cancer all the time. These stories, however, have mostly been shared from other perspectives such as by parents, health professionals, or public relations personnel, or by survivors years later; these stories are rarely ever told by the children who experience cancer themselves. I became determined to fill this void: to make space for youth with cancer to tell their own stories.

For my Honors thesis in English,[1] I sat down beside children between the ages of 8 and 21, encouraging each patient to express what it is like living with cancer. Through verbal conversations, written texts, and/or visual representations, these youth with cancer shared with me their personal and intimate experiences. With the support of Dr. Rajen Mody, a Mott pediatric oncologist and Principal Investigator for this research, and Professor Melanie Yergeau, my thesis advisor from the U-M Department of English, this idea has grown into so much more than I could ever have hoped.

---

[1] Available online at: http://deepblue.lib.umich.edu/handle/2027.42/107767

I greatly appreciate the financial and overall support that made this research possible from the University of Michigan Department of English, the LSA Honors Program, and the Division of Pediatric Hematology/Oncology. I also want to thank Jasna Markovac with the University of Michigan Medical School Learning Program, for she encouraged my publishing ambitions and devoted a great deal of time to make this book a reality. All proceeds from this book received by the Division of Pediatric Hematology/Oncology will be donated: 50% to the Block Out Cancer campaign for pediatric cancer research at the University of Michigan and 50% to the Child and Family Life Program at C.S. Mott Children's Hospital.

It has been an honor to listen to these children, to give them a chance to have their voice be heard. The following written and drawn narratives illuminate aspects of childhood cancer that too often remain hidden. Lexie, Mary, William, Shannon, Celeste, Jacob, Tamia, Zoey, Christina, and Ruben provide insight into the unique intricacies to each of their cancer experiences. My hope is that their stories will be a resource for all those involved with childhood cancer. Only in appreciating these unique experiences, I believe, can we work together to treat the many facets of cancer.

The people at C. S. Mott Children's Hospital— from physicians, nurses, and child life specialists to parents, siblings, and patients— have all inspired me to cherish these children and devote myself to their cause. As an aspiring pediatric oncologist, I want to dedicate my life to these children, to someday confront childhood cancer with compassion.

My heartfelt gratitude goes out to Mott families, whose encouragement has always meant so much to me. Most importantly, I am grateful to the children at Mott. It has truly been a privilege to spend time getting to know these youth with cancer over the years. In sharing part of their lives with me, these children have touched my own life. Now, it is my honor to share their stories with you.

Trisha Paul, B.S.
University of Michigan Medical School

CHAPTER 1

Lexie, age 15

TEENS TAKING OUT CANCER

By: Lexie

Devastating Diagnosis

Devastating, horrifying, and heart-breaking are some of the most common words associated with the word cancer. Although being diagnosed with cancer is a hard thing to deal with and understand, it doesn't have to be that bad especially if you have a good attitude about it. That is what I am here for; to share my personal experience and to answer the many frequently asked questions. Hopefully, this will give teens a better understanding of how this whole "cancer" things works.

Q.) What was it like to be diagnosed?

A.) Being diagnosed was hard, all my friends and family were crushed. Unfortunately, I have been diagnosed 5 times so for me, after a while, the words "you have cancer" didn't really faze me.

Q.) How did you feel when you were diagnosed?

A.) Like I said before, hearing that I had cancer didn't really faze me. Generally, I have a pretty upbeat attitude about things. Of course I was sad, but I knew sort of what was going to happen; I faced the facts and moved on.

Q.) How did you tell your friends about your diagnosis?

A.) Telling my friends was always a challenge. It was hard explaining that I wouldn't be able to go out or join in on parties, that I would be sick and tired most of the time, that they wouldn't see me at school very much. Lucky for me, all of my friends really understood; they tried to comfort me and told me no matter what we would still be friends.

Stupid Symptoms

Everyone's symptoms vary depending on medication and treatment plans. Some symptoms can be as little as headaches, stomach aches, soreness and fatigue. More serious stuff could be skin rashes and other skin issues, organ issues bone thinning and all kinds of other stuff, but don't let that worry you everyone is different just be prepared for what could happen.

Q.) What is cancer?

A.) Cancer can be represented in many ways. Sarcomas and Lymphomas are two common types of cancers. Within those two categories there are tons of different types of cancer, some are tumors, some are skin, some are organ or they could be like mine, blood cancer.

Q.) What does cancer look like?

A.) Cancer can be seen many different ways. Pale skin, skinny faces, bumps or rashes, bald heads, handi-cap, even amputees. Nevertheless, we are still people and that is how we should be treated.

Q.) What do you like or not like about your cancer?

A.) Well, there are many things I like and don't like about having cancer, One thing I like is all the great people I've befriended and experiences I've gotten to see, but there are many things I have had to miss out on due to appointments or just not feeling well.

A Home at the Hospital

You will find that the hospital becomes your second home and the staff your second family. It is pretty easy to assume that you will be in and out of the hospital a lot. Medicine does funny things to your body and sometime they bring you in for a fever or other things. If you plan for the stay and bring things to keep you busy, the stays are really not that bad.

Q.) What do you like about being in the hospital/ what don't you like?

A.) I probably speak for most of the patients when I say the best part about being in the hospital is the 24/7 attention and care and upbeat nurses. What isn't the best is the below average food, the IV pumps constantly going off and the late night interruptions.

Q.) What do you do when you are in the hospital?

A.) I try to do as much as I can while I feel good, but because the medicines made me feel tired and icky and the pumps kept me up all night I didn't really feel up to doing a whole lot. I am not sure about other hospitals, but U of M offers art therapy, music therapy, a wonderful child-life program that can assist you with crafts, games or just someone to hang out with; also they have pizza and live entertainment on Thursday night for the people who are in-patient.

Tricky Treatments and Tips to Getting Through

Depending on what type of cancer or where it is in your body, treatment plans can vary greatly. In my personal experience I've had a variety of different treatments. I've had radiation, many different types of chemo therapy, and a bone marrow transplant and now we are starting a new therapy called Immunotherapy. It's pretty safe to say that I have seen almost all of it. During my long life of cancer I have learned the tricks and trades of making it through. There are some really simple things that you can do to make a crappy day a little better. (Look in the back for some fun tips and tricks)

Q.) What are some things you like about being treated/ what are some things you don't like?

A.) Well, I can't say that there is a whole lot of things I like about being treated other than the fact that it is keeping my cancer at bay. Certainly, I can tell you a lot of things I don't like. One thing I don't like is how chemo and other treatments make me feel. Sometimes they make me feel icky and tired almost all the time. The one thing I hate the most though is the time spent away from friends. You may find yourself alone at times because your friends don't ask you to hang out. My advice, don't get mad at them or blame them for not hanging out with you because that could stir up a lot of problems. Most of the time they don't know how to react, chances are they really want to be your friend still.

Q.) How did you/ do you keep your spirits up during treatment?

A.) This question is my most frequently asked question; it's like everyone wants to know my secret or something. Here is the thing, cancer sucks and we all know it so instead of wasting the little energy I have left pouting and throwing myself a pity party, why not smile and try to enjoy life a little. I find that if I keep a more positive attitude my appointments go faster, treatments feel better and in general people want to be around me more.

A Teens Advice

Throughout my journey with cancer I have experienced a lot. There were many things I wish I never knew about, but there have been many experiences that I am very grateful I have been able to take part in. If I could give anyone advice the biggest piece of advice I can give is to have a good attitude and try to live life to the best of your ability because later on you will regret all the opportunities you passed up.

Q.) What advice would you give to a teen that has just been diagnosed?

A.) My advice to any teen that has just been diagnosed is to live life like nothing is going on. Don't pass opportunities up because you don't think you can do something or are too embarrassed. Nothing about cancer is positive, but you can make the best out of the situation. For a long time I didn't want to swim in front of my friends because I couldn't wear a wig in the pool. Just recently I was at a friend's birthday party and it was a bowling party but I had a fractured foot so I didn't think I could play. My friends were so supportive; they even helped me bowl so I could join in on the fun! I would have never known how much fun either of these things would have been if I had let silly little embarrassments get in my way. Another piece of advice is to speak up. If you don't like something or something doesn't feel right you need to say something. It is so important for you to voice your opinion because the doctors and nurses can sometimes fix things to make them more comfortable, and remember they are human too they could have made a mistake.

Q.) What kind of things do you want adults in your life to know about what it's like to have cancer?

A.) I assumed they meant adults in general when they asked this question. I want them all to know that we are just normal kids; we don't need to be talked to differently, looked at funny, asked embarrassing questions and monitored like prey every minute. This goes for family, friends, people in public and doctors.

Remember and Reflect

When reflecting back on my journey only one question is asked that's really important. It's basically two questions in one but it has such a huge impact.

Q.) Has cancer changed your life and would you change it all if you could?

A.) I am not sure I would change everything. Cancer has been a part of my life for so long, it has made me who I am and allowed me to see things in a whole different way. If I were to change anything about my cancer it would be the amount of relapses. One time through is more than anyone should have to deal with, 5 times is not something I have enjoyed.

Cancer has made me realize that life isn't easy, but you have to have faith, trust and courage; with these three things, you can accomplish anything! The journey, as awful as it is has shown me to go for my dreams and work extra hard because I have been given the gift of life and I can't waist something so precious. Currently, I have my own non-profit organization that aids sick children and children in poverty. I am an honors student and I have a job working with young children, Yes, I still take chemo, but I try really hard to run as normal of a life as possible.

A Few Facts about Me!

Now that we have gotten through all the questions and stuff I am sure you are curious as to who wrote this. Well, my name is Lexie and I am an only child. I live at home with two dogs and cat, which I love very much. Some of my favorite hobbies are crafting, swimming, writing, spending time with friends and watching movies. A few of my favorite TV shows are Criminal Minds, Full House, George Lopez, cooking competitions and the Style Network. Normally, I am a pretty busy person; I have tutored for elementary age reading, I work at a pre-school and I run a non- profit organization. When I am not busy with any of that I try to spend time with family and friends.

Now that you have gotten to know a little bit about me and have read my experiences and thoughts, I hope that your questions and worries have been clarified. Hopefully, you enjoyed my story and are inspired to get out and live life, work for your dreams and get out of your comfort zone.

Thanks for reading!

Lexie

IDEAS, TIPS AND TRICKS!

Easy hospital food treats

Creamsicles in a cup:

. 1 single serving of orange sherbet (raspberry works well too)

. 1 single serving of vanilla ice cream

- Scoop both into cup and mix until soft, then ENJOY!

Sunday breakfast scramble (close enough)

.Order of scrambled eggs

.Order of link sausage or hot dog

.1 slice of cheese (your preference)

- Slice sausage and mix in with eggs. Place cheese on top and microwave for 30 seconds.
- Enjoy!

Crafts and other fun ideas!

. Practice your skills by solving crossword puzzles and other mind games

. Start a blog or write in a journal

. Build a model car or paint a pot

. Knit a scarf

. Make make-up, hair or nail tutorials

. Create fan pages or interest pages on Facebook

. Write a song or poem

Fun, safe websites for all age's not just teens!

- http://www.imvu.com (recommended for teens only)
- http://www.howrse.com
- http://www.stardoll.com/en
- http://www.edheads.org
- www.coolmath-games.com
- http://pbskids.org/games/
- http://disneychannel.disney.com/games
- http://www.barbie.com/activities/fun_games/#/whats-hot
- http://www.miniclip.com/games/en

CHAPTER 2

Mary, age 13

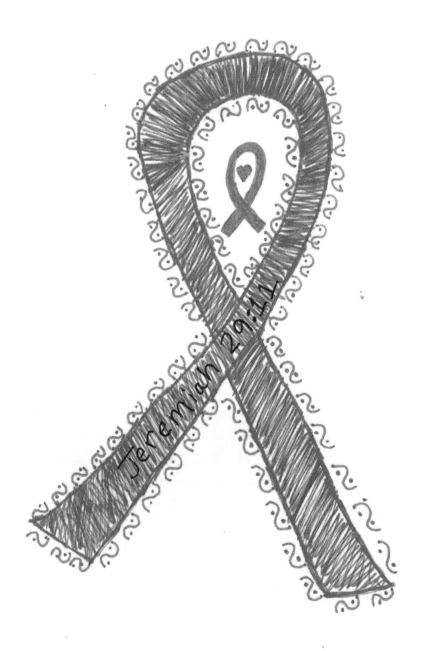

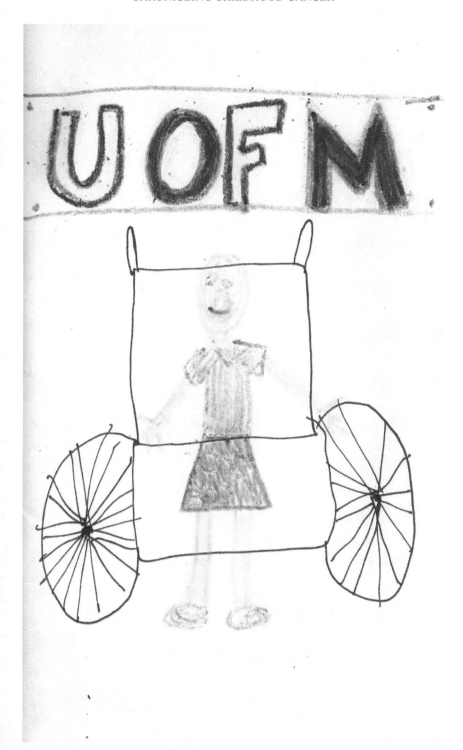

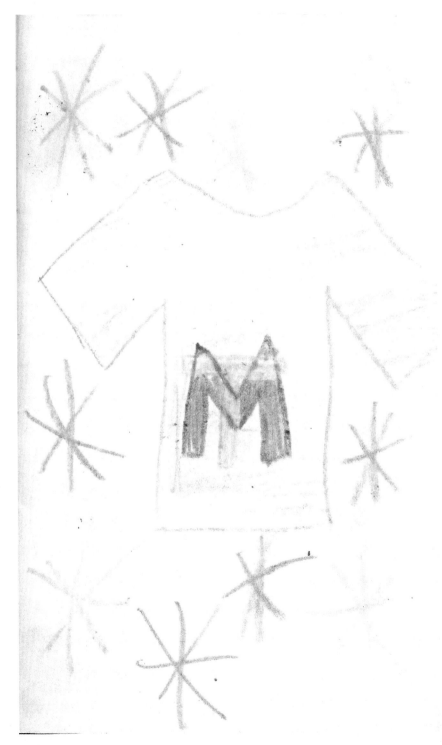

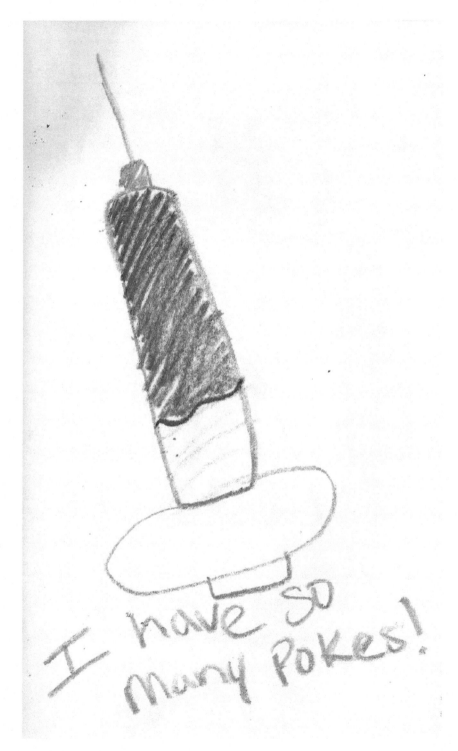

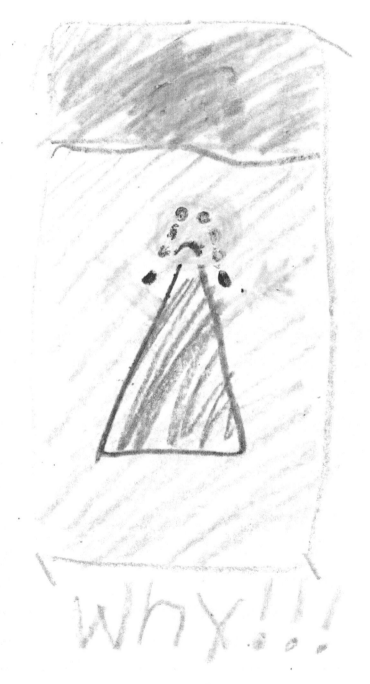

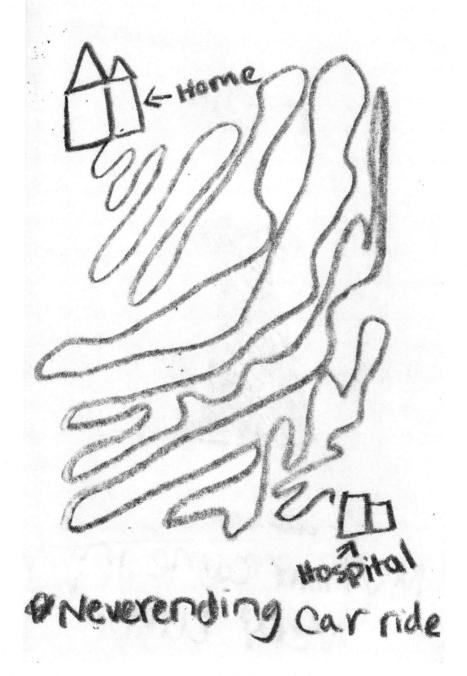

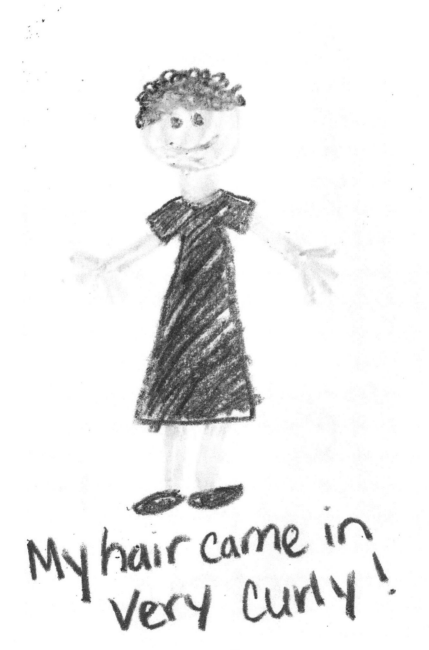

My hair came in very curly!

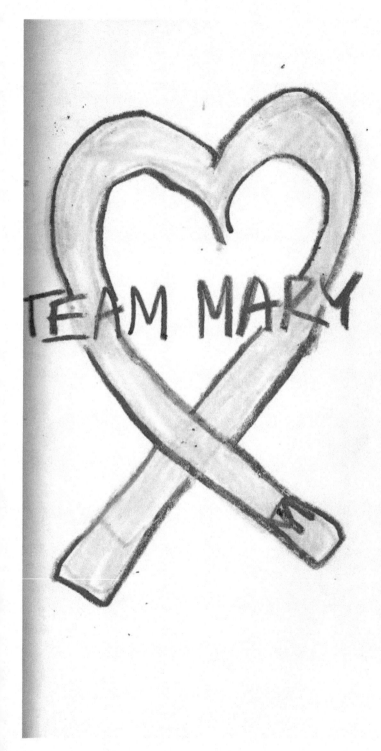

CHAPTER 3

William, age 11

1. Diagnosis
- sad
- upset
- DIE
- Can't do a lot of things
- Frustrated

2. Symptoms
- Disavantange
- Bad blood cells
- Good Treatment
- Don't like being in the Hospital
- Don't like missing school
- Medicine STINKS!

- Cancer makes me feel sad

- Hospital
- Sick at school
- lot of tooth bleeds
- urgent care
  saint.JOSe
  childrens mott
- Sleeping a lot
- Activity room
- Atheles
- ~~so~~ dont like food
- ~~me~~   dont like

Medicine

- makes ~~food~~ ~~taste~~ taste nasty
- missing family, school
  friend
- Play Games
- watch tv
- Arts and crarts

- Treatment
- kimo
- radiation
- sad
- Tired
- makes me sick

Like that chemo makes
you get well

spirits ↑
watch TV
Play Games
Listen to music

Advice

. The Nurse will treat
you well. Know that
it will be okay. Don't
feel sad or down.

-Cancer-
If a person

Treat the cancer well
dont be mean to it

-Adults to know-
I don't like it... it feels
hard... its Hard.

Reflection -

No! I can still do a lot of stuff.

I like doing the videos for UofM and make-a-wish

CHAPTER 4

Shannon, age 12

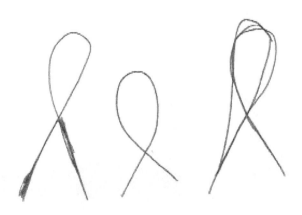

My Chemo
Journey

by. Shannon

Blood
Draw.

The first start of
chemo is
Blood draw.

Me , shelia

mom

Doctor Visit

The second step of chemo is the doctor visit.

(Shannon)

mom

2

Chemo lab. The third step is getting my treatment.

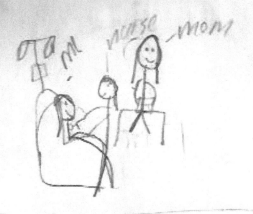

Child life

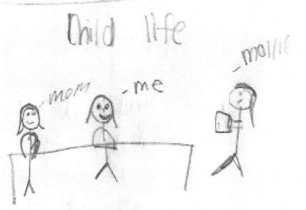

During my treatments you can go to the child life room.

3

friends at chemo with me.

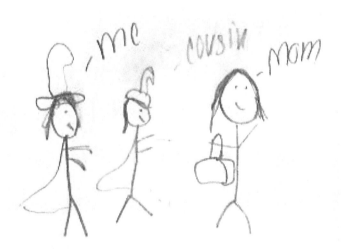

One time at chemo I brought my cousin and wi wire allowed to dress up.

4

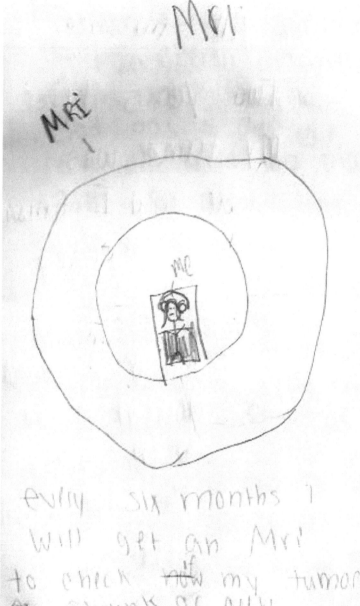

evriy six months I
will get an Mri
to check how my tumor
if shrunk or grew.

5

All finished.

Two years later
My tumor was
stable and I finished
Chemo Therapy.

After I finished
chemo. I started
Volleyball and
been going
to school full
time.

Having cancer stinks!
Having chemo stinks
even more! However,
God has a plan for
everyone and His plan
was for me to have
a tumor. His plan
was for me to
have chemo for
two years. I don't
understand why but
I have faith that
God knows what He
is doing and I Hope
I am done with
being sick. I thank
God for putting so many
wonderful people in the
path of my chemo
Journey.

CHAPTER 5

Celeste, age 17

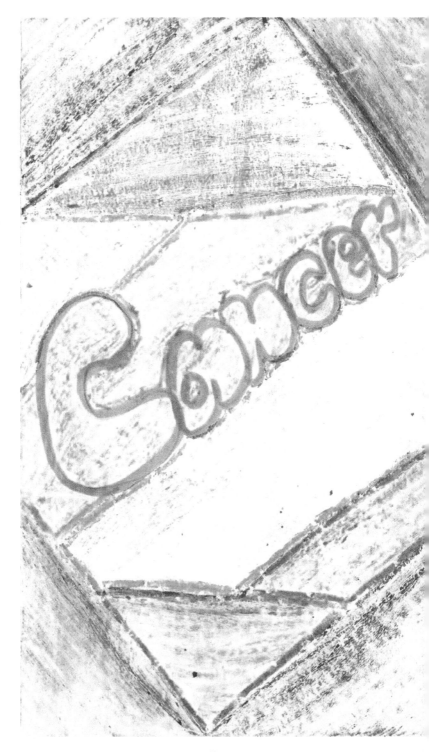

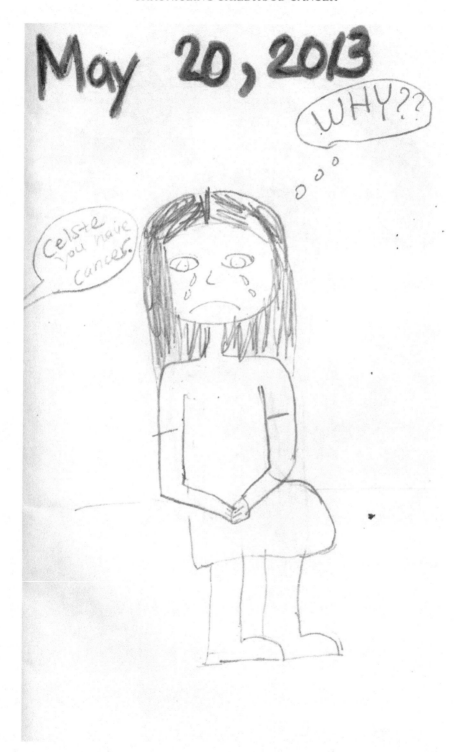

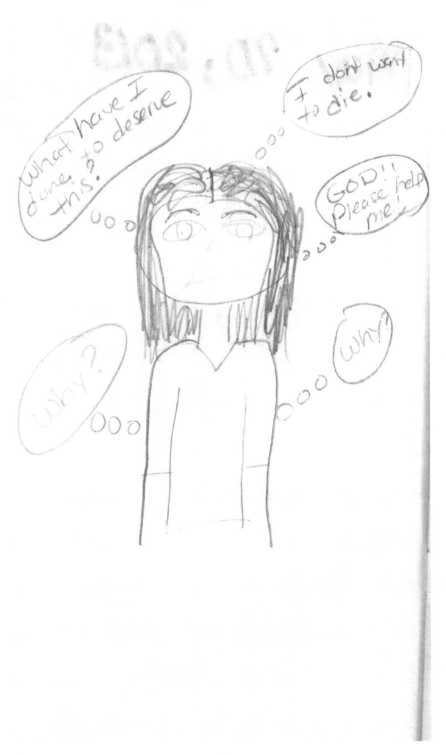

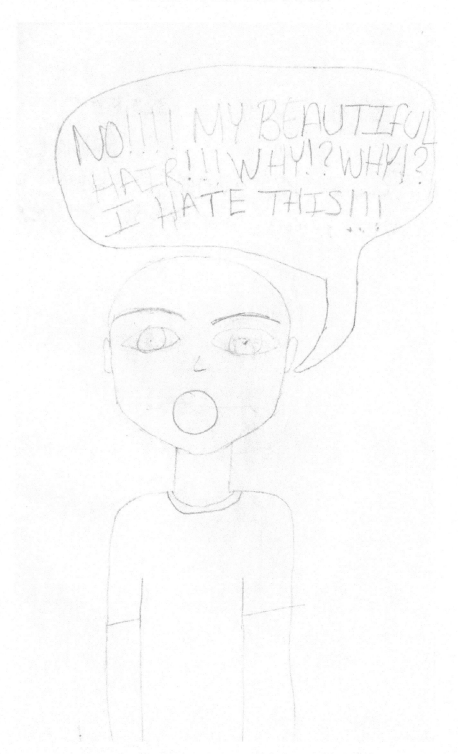

I'm sorry for putting all of you in this situation, sorry for having you change your plans because of me.

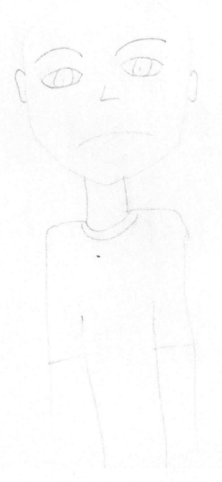

All these smells are making me nauseous...
I am gonna throw up.

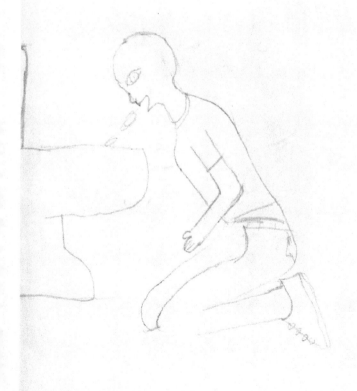

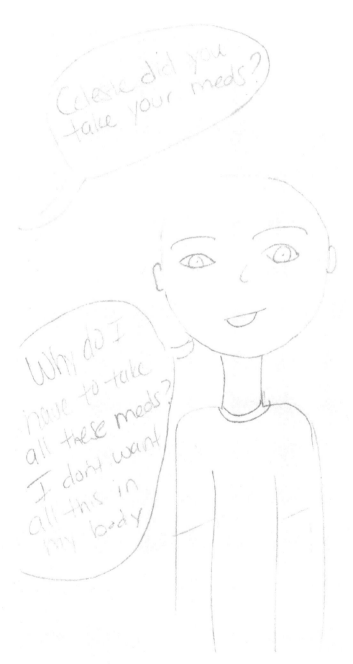

MY Medicine

Colace for constipation

Reglan for nausea and
vomitting

Adavan for nausea and
vomitting

Antibiotic for protection
against infections.

Miralax for constipation

Ibuprofen for pain and
swelling.

I have learned to accept the fact that I have Cancer and I want to get threw this therapy.

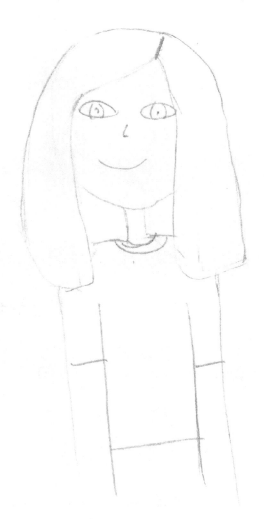

CHAPTER 6

Jacob, age 15

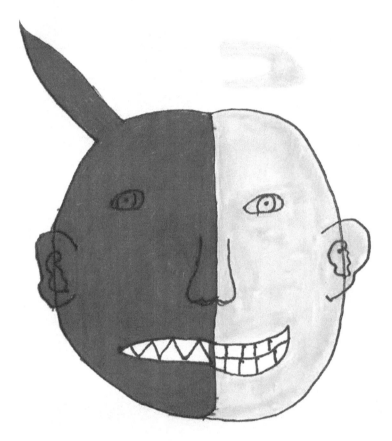

Cancer is half and half.
It can be the devil, or
it can be angle. It
all depends on your
attitude.

1. It was scary to be diagnosed.
2. same ↗
3. By the time I woke up from intiba-
and got back home, the whole town tion
knew about it.

4. Cells the grow to fast.
5.
6. The treaments.
7. tired and sick.
8. I couldnt breath.
9. People are nice.
10. watch tv, Play games, walk around.

11. chemo
12. Tired and sick.
13. It takes your cancer away.
14. #12

15. My Parents, but mainly it's the mind set you have. Don't let yourself think that.

16. Thank you, and hate you.
17. Keep your head up and don't let it get to you.

18. ~~I~~ Nobody wants to be treated like a baby.

19. Yes, I've gotten to do so much more than normal, and it made me appreciate things in life more.

ALWAYS KEEP YOUR HEAD UP!
It could be worse!

CHAPTER 7

Tamia, age 14

Being diagnosed with
Cancer isnt easy. Me And
my family were going threw
a very hard time. Lots
of sadness, And everyone
was very worried About me.

It didnt feel good to be
diagnosed with Cancer, I
was very upset And scared.

When I told my friends
I had cancer, I just
came out And told them
threw text message. Most
of my friends couldnt believe
it.

Cancer is tumors. Some Are big, some are small.

It looks like circles. I've never really saw A tumor, but I'm guessing it can come in all shapes, And sizes.

I dont really like Anything about CANCER. I hate Everything about it.

CANCER makes me feel horrible. It causes lots of pain.

I went to the Hospital
in Nashville, because I was
having trouble breathing,
And swallowing my food.

I like the Nurses, And
Doctors At the hospital. Thats
really the only reason I
would be happy to go
there.

I dont like being in the hospital
because sometimes I have
to get chemo, And I dont
really like to be alone while
Im there. So Im always
trying to get Someone out
here to see me.

When I'm at the hospital,
usually, I would just stay
in my room, watch t.v, or
play on my IPad.
And sometimes I would
go down to the play room,
and mahe something.

To treat my cancer I am
getting lots of chemo. I
was getting radiation, but I
finished that in June. ☺
Treatment mahes me feel
very weah and tired.
Sometimes it even mahes
my emotions go all over the
place. One minute I'm
happy, the next I'm upset,
and crying, or very mad
and annoyed.

I dont like Anything about being treated. It all really sucks. With being so weak and tired, you dont feel like doing anything but sleeping, And lying in bed. And its really hard to do anything by yourself. You always need help.

I dont really know how I keep my spirt up. Its really hard for me. Most of the time I fake A smile And act like Im doing fine. Mostly because I dont want my family or friends to worry about me.

If cancer was a person.
I would probably ask it
why is it give this to us,
~~and~~ And weve done nothing
to them. Its ~~tatting~~ peoples
lives, And it just isnt fair.
Id probably pray that
Cancer gets cancer and
dies.

If your a kid or ~~adult~~ adult
thats going threw cancer
just know this. It may
be hard, but if you believe
in yourself, And dont give
up, you'll make it threw.
Your Stronger than any
illness.

I could try to talk to the
Adults in my life, And tell
them how hard it is, but
really, they will never
understand it.

I guess this is the kind
of thing you have to go
threw in order to understand
it.
Cancer has changed my
life a lot. Me and my family
has goten a lot closer, and
I've leared a lot. I think
Im more respectful, and
thought ful than I was
before.
I've had lots of ups, and
downs in my life, but
I believe I have a
great future ahead of me.
And there is no way Im
going to let cancer take
me away.

CHAPTER 8

Zoey, age 9

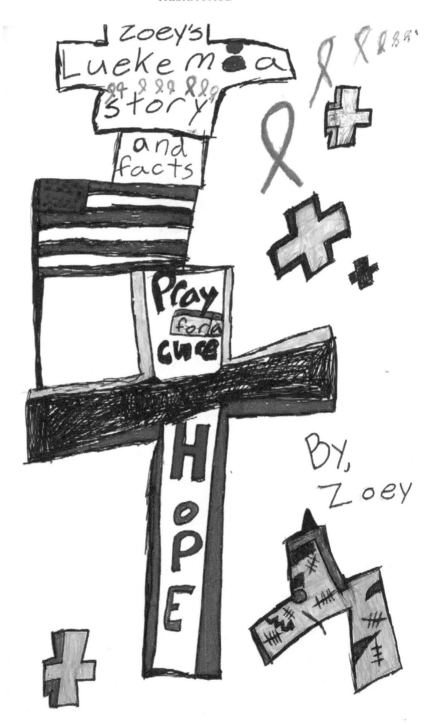

What was it like to be diagnosed? It was sad to leave Home.

How did I feel to tell my friends I was diagnosed? Sad "!!!!!

Facts about cancer

Whats cancer? well it just comes and goes.

How cancer makes me feel? weak.

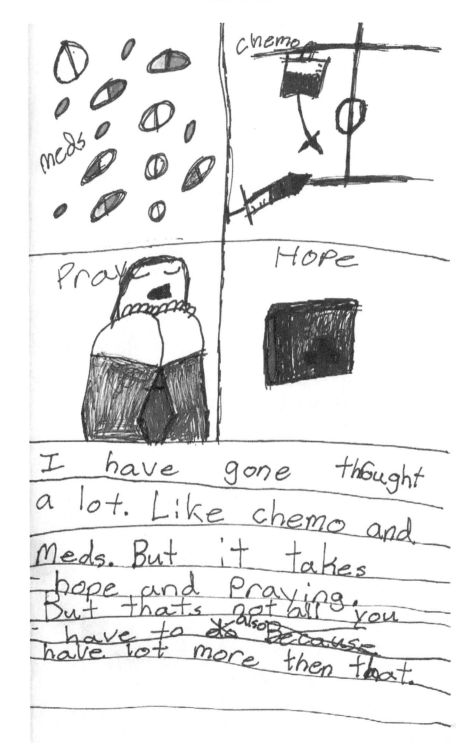

I have gone thought a lot. Like chemo and Meds. But it takes hope and praying. But thats not all you have to do also Because have lot more then that.

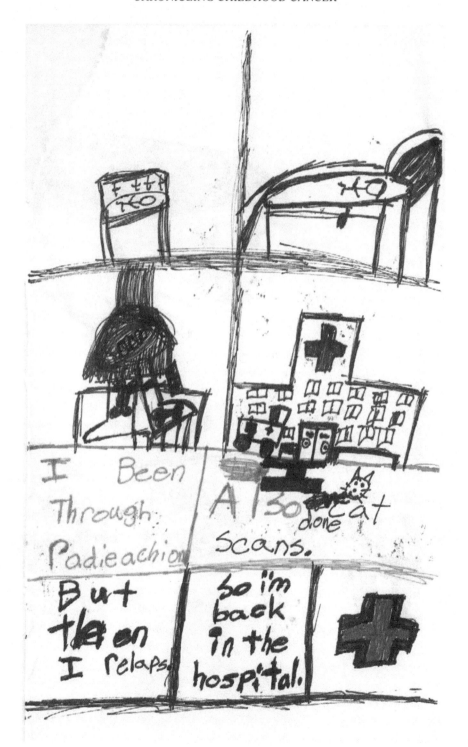

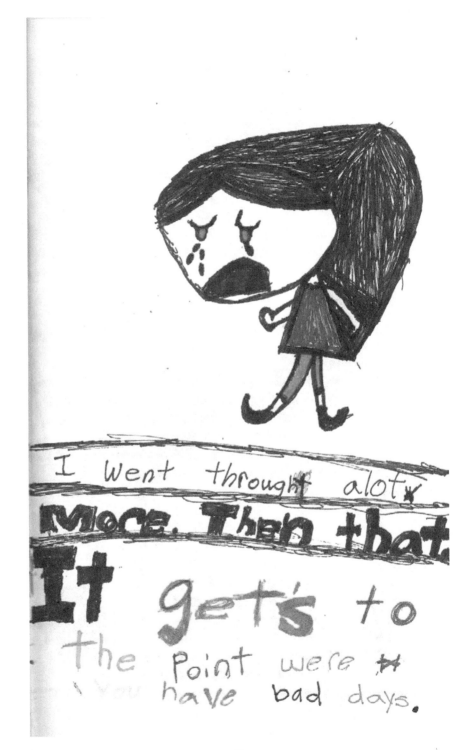

I went through alot. More. Then that It get's to the Point were it you have bad days.

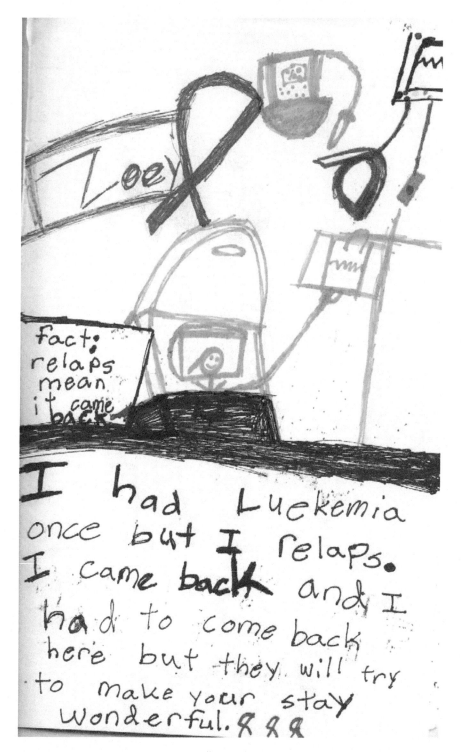

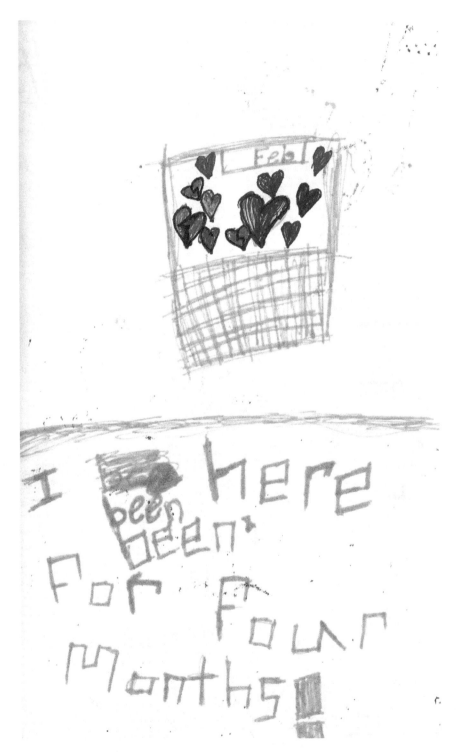

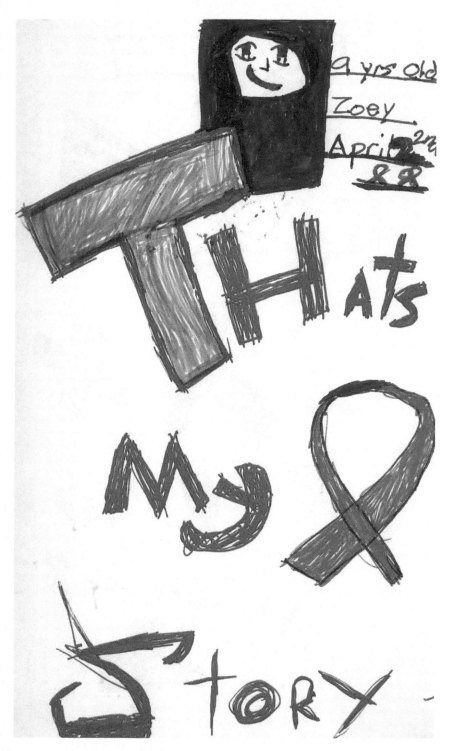

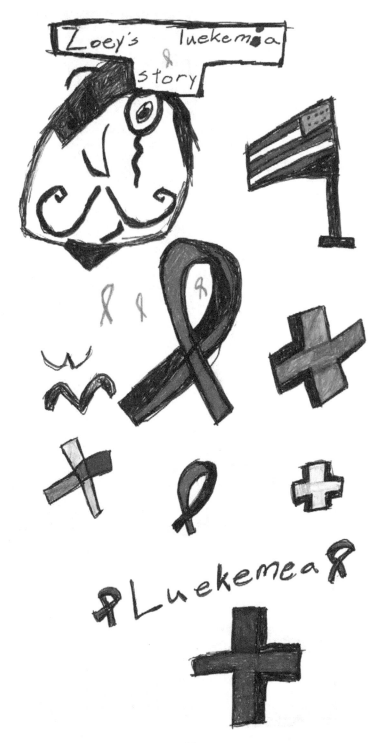

CHAPTER 9

Christina, age 16

My Story........

Hi, My name is Christina and I live in Detroit, MI and this is my story. I guess I should start from the beginning. When I was 2 weeks old I was diagnosed with Crohnes disease (I.B.S - Irritable Bowel Syndrome) and ever since then I had serious stomach issues that effected my whole life such like my Height, Weight, and more. Over the years I grew up differently than other kids. When I was first born I Spent the first 5 Years of my life in the Hospital. Ever since then I've been In and out of the Hospital constantly for the past 16 years for Appointments, and Most of the time in the Emergency room. Then when I was 10 My Doctor of 14 years prescribed me with HUMIRA. I took it for 2 years until one day I couldn't eat anything without getting sick. I didn't have the normal appetite like I usually have. I was so tired even though I got enough sleep before I went to school that day. I thought maybe I had pneumonia like I always have in the past. Then my stomach was really red and bloated. I was just about to end my

1st semester of 7th grade at Hoover Middle School in Taylor. So since I wasn't feeling any good, my parents picked me from school and took me to the emergency room. And then I got admitted. A couple days later after doing a lot of tests my Dad came into my room trying to hold his tears in and he said that I had "Cancer." It was Lymphoma. My parents told me that I got it from an allergic reaction to the HUMIRA that I took for the past 2 years. The BEST part of it is that it was treatable and I was ganna live. The Docs said that we caught the tumor in time before It got even worse. A week later I started treatment. It took 2-3 weeks for my hair to fall off but I got through it well. After 9 Months - 1 year of treatment I was cured. Even though it was a very hard, long, and painful ride I got through it with my Family and friends. After 2 years of Remission. Going to lots of scans, and lots of Check Ups. I thought everything was going swell and ok. My hair finally grew back, I got to see my friends again, I graduated middle school in Honors, I got through Freshman year in Truman High School. Until......... I came in for my next scan that was planned every 2 months. I thought it was okay and it was normal until. The Docs found something. At first I was terrified of what it was. So they ordered a Biopsy and the results came back Positive for Cancer sells. I thought when I first heard it from my dad that he was joking (Because he plays around with me) and then he started crying. And I knew that was bad because he never cries unless it really hurts. At first I kept repeating "Please be Joking" on and on and on until finally I broke down and started balling my eyes out. Then I knew it was true. I had Cancer the thing that changed my life. The thing I never thought I would have again. I told my Best Friend/Sister Raven about it and just like I was we were both crying on the phone trying to understand what we're saying. Then we finally calmed down and I told her "I start Chemo next Week". So I go in the week after to get a Line put in for my Chemo. And I start Chemo the next day. Ever since that hard couple weeks things have cooled down a little. I went 2 school for a couple days then I went for a whole month. Then the best news I've been hoping for my whole life. The thing that can cure my Cancer and my Crohnes for good. The best I can explain it is it's a Bone Marrow Transplant. I don't know who the Donor is but I'm excited to meet Him/Her. What they do is they give me another line which I'm Getting put in this Wednesday. I'm also Ganna be getting more Chemo and then I'm Ganna be in the hospital for the whole month. After that I'm hopefully it finally cured my Cancer and my Crohnes. Now I can go on and on about My history and the Hell I went through but I will make this story as little as I can without making a book out of it. I hope this is the end of the trail I'm heading to for the rest of these couple months. The Highway to Hell I've been going on ever since I was a newborn.

CHAPTER 10

Ruben, age 13

My name is Ruben
I am the third child of three.
When I was nine I began to
feel very sick. It began with
my neck hurting to where I could
not move it. Later the pain
went down to my chest and ribs.
My mom took me to see my Pediatrician
Docter Natasha Umlauf who tested
my blood and when my resolts came in
She told my mom to take me to UofM.
when I arrived I told the docter
what I was feeling. Latr came
back and told my parents that I
have ALL. My mom and dad were sad
and I was scared. I went through
chemo therapy where I would get sick
and I also lost my hair. I lost weight
but today I am cancer free, I am a
Survivur, I give thanks to the steoff
and dockers of UofM for my recovery.

/ May the Lord continue to work with the docters of UofM and bless them on thire jobs everyday.

By
Ruben

WRITING ACTIVITY

The following questions were provided to encourage the narrative expressions included in this book.

1. Diagnosis
> What was it like to be diagnosed?
> How did you feel when you were diagnosed?
> How did you tell your friends about your diagnosis?

2. Symptoms
> What is cancer?
> What does cancer look like?
> What do you like or not like about your cancer?
> How does cancer make you feel?

3. Hospital
> Why did you come to the hospital?
> What do you like about being in the hospital?
> What don't you like about being in the hospital?
> What do you do when you are in the hospital?

4. Treatment
> What is being done to treat the cancer?
> How does treatment make you feel?
> What are some things that you like about being treated?
> What are some things that you don't like about being treated?
> How did you keep your spirits up during treatment?

5. Advice

If cancer was a person, what would you say or do to cancer?

What advice would you give to a child who has just been diagnosed with cancer?

What kind of things would you want the adults in your life (doctors, nurses, parents, etc.) to know about what it's like to have cancer?

6. Reflections

Has cancer changed your life? If so, how?

Anything else you would like to share about your story of the cancer experience?

TELL YOUR STORY

Are you interested in sharing your experiences with cancer? By telling your story, you can help health professionals, parents, and others to better understand what it is like to have cancer. Sharing your story may also help other children and teens with cancer like you.

We are looking for children, teens, and young adults with cancer to submit their personal story for future publications of *Chronicling Childhood Cancer: A Collection of Personal Stories by Children and Teens with Cancer.*

If you are interested in this potential opportunity to share your story, please contact the editor:

Trisha Paul

tkpaul@umich.edu

ABOUT THE EDITOR

Trisha Paul is a first year medical student at the University of Michigan Medical School. She has been volunteering with pediatric oncology patients at C.S. Mott Children's Hospital for five years, and she aspires to become a pediatric oncologist. She received a B.S. in English with Honors along with minors in Biochemistry and Medical Anthropology from the University of Michigan. Trisha writes about her experiences in literature and medicine at illnessnarratives.com.

Made in the USA
Coppell, TX
26 September 2023